# Vegetarian Diet Cookbook for Beginners

A Beginner's Guide To Healthy And Easy Vegetarian Recipes To Satisfy Any Craving And Live Better

## Natalie Clark

# Table Of Content

# Breakfast

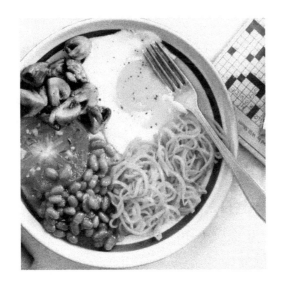

# Onion & Mushroom Tart with a Nice Brown Rice Crust

Preparation time 10 minutes

Cooking time 55 minutes

Serving: 1

Ingredients:

1 ½ pounds, mushrooms, button, portabella,

1 cup, short-grain brown rice

2 ¼ cups, water

½ teaspoon, ground black pepper

2 teaspoons, herbal spice blend

1 sweet large onion

7 ounces, extra-firm tofu

1 cup, plain non-dairy milk

2 teaspoons, onion powder

2 teaspoons, low-sodium soy

1 teaspoon, molasses

¼ teaspoon, ground turmeric

¼ cup, white wine

¼ cup, tapioca

Directions:

Cook the brown rice and put it aside for later use.

Slice the onions into thin strips and sauté them in water until they are soft. Then, add the molasses, and cook them for a few minutes.

Next, sauté the mushrooms in water with the herbal spice blend. Once the mushrooms are cooked and they are soft, add the white wine or sherry. Cook everything for a few more minutes.

In a blender, combine milk, tofu, arrowroot, turmeric, and onion powder till you have a smooth mixture

On a pie plate, create a layer of rice, spreading evenly to form a crust. The rice should be warm and not cold. It will be easy to work with warm rice. You can also use a pastry roller to get an even crust. With your fingers, gently press the sides.

Take half of the tofu mixture and the mushrooms and spoon them over the tart dish. Smooth the level with your spoon.

Now, top the layer with onions followed by the tofu mixture. You can smooth the surface again with your spoon.

Sprinkle some black pepper on top.

Bake the pie at 3500 F for about 45 minutes. Toward the end, you can cover it loosely with tin foil. This will help the crust to remain moist.

Allow the pie crust to cool down, so that you can slice it. If you are in love with vegetarian dishes, there is no way that you will not love this pie.

Nutrition: Calories: 245.3, Fats 16.4 g, Proteins 6.8 g, Carbohydrates 18.3 g

# Yogurt with Beets & Raspberries

Preparation Time: 5 minutes

Cooking Time: 0 minute

Servings: 1


Ingredients:

1 cup soy yogurt

½ cup beets, cooked and sliced

1 tablespoon raspberry jam

1 tablespoon almonds, slivered


Directions:

Mix all the ingredients in a glass jar with lid.

Sprinkle the almonds on top.

Refrigerate for up to 2 days.

Nutrition: Calories: 281 Total fat: 7.3g Saturated fat: 2.7g

Cholesterol: 15mg Sodium: 237mg Potassium: 882mg

Carbohydrates: 40.2g Fiber: 2.5g Sugar: 36g Protein: 15.7g

# Curry Oatmeal

Preparation Time: 10 minutes

Cooking Time: 0 minute

Servings: 3


Ingredients:

1 tablespoon pure peanut butter

½ cup rolled oats

½ cup coconut milk

½ teaspoon curry powder

1 teaspoon tamari

¼ cup cooked kale

1 tablespoon cilantro, chopped

2 tablespoons tomatoes, chopped


Directions:

Mix all the ingredients except the kale, cilantro and tomatoes.

Transfer to a glass jar with lid.

Refrigerate for up to 5 days.

Top with the remaining ingredients when ready to serve.

Nutrition: Calories: 307 Total fat: 13.8g Saturated fat: 4g

Cholesterol: 12mg Sodium: 467mg Potassium: 890mg

Carbohydrates: 34.1g Fiber: 3g Sugar: 2g Protein: 10.1g

# Breakfast Cherry Delight

Preparation time: 10 minutes

Cooking time: 8 hours and 10 minutes

Servings: 4


Ingredients:

2 cups almond milk

2 cups water

1 cup steel cut oats

2 tablespoons cocoa powder

1/3 cup cherries, pitted

¼ Cup maple syrup

½ Teaspoon almond extract

For the sauce:

2 tablespoons water

1 and ½ cups cherries, pitted and chopped

¼ Teaspoon almond extract


Directions:

Put the almond milk in your slow cooker.

Add 2 cups water, oats, cocoa powder, 1/3 cup cherries, maples syrup and ½ teaspoon almond extract.

Stir, cover and cook on low for 8 hours.

In a small pan, mix 2 tablespoons water with 1 and ½ cups cherries and ¼ teaspoon almond extract, stir well, bring to a simmer over medium heat and cook for 10 minutes until it thickens.

Divide oatmeal into breakfast bowls, top with the cherries sauce and serve.

Enjoy!

Nutrition: calories 150, fat 1, fiber 2, carbs 6, protein 5

# Perfect Breakfast Shake

Preparation time: 5 minutes

Cooking time: 0 minutes

Servings: 2


Ingredients:

3 tablespoons, raw cacao powder

1 cup, almond milk

2 frozen bananas

3 tablespoons, natural peanut butter


Directions:

Use a powerful blender to combine all the ingredients.

Process everything until you have a smooth shake.

Enjoy a hearty shake to kickstart your day.

Nutrition: Calories: 330, Fats 15 g, Carbohydrates 41 g, Proteins 11 g

# Hearty French Toast Bowls

Preparation time: 10 minutes

Cooking time: 5 hours

Servings: 4

Ingredients:

1 and ½ cups almond milk

1 cup coconut cream

1 tablespoon vanilla extract

½ Tablespoon cinnamon powder

2 tablespoons maple syrup

¼ Cup spenda

2 apples, cored and cubed

½ Cup cranberries, dried

1 pound vegan bread, cubed

Cooking spray

Directions: Spray your slow cooker with some cooking spray and add the bread. Also, add cranberries and apples and stir gently. Add milk, coconut cream, maple syrup, vanilla extract, cinnamon powder and splenda. Stir, cover and cook on low for 5 hours. Divide into bowls and serve right away. Enjoy!

Nutrition: calories 140, fat 2, fiber 3, carbs 6, protein 2

# Peanut Butter Granola

Preparation time: 10 minutes

Cooking time: 47 minutes

Servings: 04


Ingredients:

Nonstick spray

4 cups oats

⅓ cup of cocoa powder

¾ cup peanut butter

⅓ cup maple syrup

⅓ cup avocado oil

1½ teaspoons vanilla extract

½ cup cocoa nibs

6 ounces dark chocolate, chopped


Directions:

Preheat your oven to 300 degrees F.

Spray a baking sheet with cooking spray.

In a medium saucepan add oil, maple syrup, and peanut butter.

Cook for 2 minutes on medium heat, stirring.

Add the oats and cocoa powder, mix well.

Spread the coated oats on the baking sheet.

---

Bake for 45 minutes, occasionally stirring.

Garnish with dark chocolate, cocoa nibs, and peanut butter. Serve.

Nutrition: Calories 134 Total Fat 4.7 g Saturated Fat 0.6 g Cholesterol 124mg Sodium 1 mg Total Carbs 54.1 g Fiber 7 g Sugar 3.3 g Protein 6.2 g

# Pumpkin Spice Bites

Preparation time: 10 minutes

Cooking time: 0 minutes

Servings: 2


Ingredients:

½ cup pumpkin puree

½ cup almond butter

¼ cup maple syrup

1 teaspoon pumpkin pie spice

1⅓ cup rolled oats

⅓ cup pumpkin seeds

⅓ cup raisins

2 tablespoons chia seeds


Directions  In a sealable container, add everything and mix well.  Seal the container and refrigerate overnight.  Roll the mixture into small balls.  Serve.

Nutrition: Calories 212 Total Fat 11.8 g Saturated Fat 2.2 g Cholesterol 23mg Sodium 321 mg Total Carbs 14.6 g Fibers 4.4 g Sugar 8 g Protein 7.3g

# Apple Chia Pudding

Preparation time: 10 minutes

Cooking time: 5 minutes

Servings: 04

Ingredients:

Chia Pudding:

4 tablespoons chia seeds

1 cup almond milk

½ teaspoon cinnamon

Apple Pie Filling:

1 large apple, peeled, cored and chopped

¼ cup water

2 teaspoons maple syrup

Pinch cinnamon

2 tablespoons golden raisins

Directions:

In a sealable container, add cinnamon, chia seeds and almond milk, mix well.

Seal the container and refrigerate overnight.

In a medium pot, combine all apple pie filling ingredients and cook for 5 minutes.

Serve the chia pudding with apple filling on top.

Enjoy.

Nutrition: Calories 387 Total Fat 5.8 g Saturated Fat 4.2 g Cholesterol 41 mg Sodium 154 mg Total Carbs 24.1 g Fiber 2.9 g Sugar 3.1 g Protein 6.6 g

# Entrées

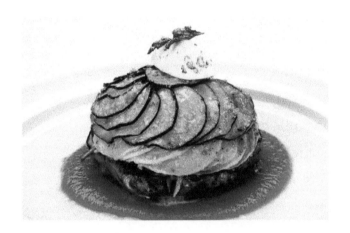

# Crazy Maple and Pear Breakfast

Preparation time: 10 minutes

Cooking time: 9 hours

Servings: 2

Ingredients:

1 pear, cored and chopped

½ Teaspoon maple extract

2 cups coconut milk

½ Cup steel cut oats

½ Teaspoon vanilla extract

1 tablespoon stevia

¼ Cup walnuts, chopped for serving

Cooking spray

Directions:

Spray your slow cooker with some cooking spray and add coconut milk.

Also, add maple extract, oats, pear, stevia and vanilla extract, stir, cover and cook on low for 9 hours.

Stir your oatmeal again, divide it into breakfast bowls and serve with chopped walnuts on top.

Enjoy!

# Cucumber Bites with Chive and Sunflower Seeds

Preparation time: 5 minutes

Cooking time: 5 minutes

Servings: 2

Ingredients:

1 cup raw sunflower seed

½ teaspoon salt

½ cup chopped fresh chives

1 clove garlic, chopped

2 tablespoons red onion, minced

2 tablespoons lemon juice

½ cup water (might need more or less)

4 large cucumbers

Directions:

Place the sunflower seeds and salt in the food processor and process to a fine powder. It will take only about 10 seconds. Add the chives, garlic, onion, lemon juice and water and process until creamy, scraping down the sides frequently. The mixture should be very creamy; if not, add a little more water. Cut the cucumbers into 1½-inch coin-like pieces.

Spread a spoonful of the sunflower mixture on top and set on a platter. Sprinkle more chopped chives on top and refrigerate until ready to serve.

# Crunchy Asparagus Spears

Preparation time: 25 minutes

Cooking time: 25 minutes

Servings: 4

Ingredients:

1 bunch asparagus spears (about 12 spears)

¼ cup nutritional yeast

2 tablespoons hemp seeds

1 teaspoon garlic powder

¼ teaspoon paprika (or more if you like paprika)

⅛ teaspoon ground pepper

¼ cup whole-wheat breadcrumbs

Juice of ½ lemon

Directions:

Preheat the oven to 350 degrees, Fahrenheit. Line a baking sheet with parchment paper.

Wash the asparagus, snapping off the white part at the bottom. Save it for making vegetable stock.

Mix together the nutritional yeast, hemp seed, garlic powder, paprika, pepper and breadcrumbs.

Place asparagus spears on the baking sheets giving them a little room in between and sprinkle with the mixture in the bowl.

Bake for up to 25 minutes, until crispy.

Serve with lemon juice if desired.

# Soups, Salads, and Sides

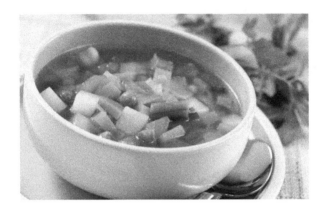

# Coconut Watercress Soup

Preparation time: 10 minutes

Cooking time: 20 minutes

Servings: 4

Ingredients:

1 teaspoon coconut oil

1 onion, diced

¾ cup coconut milk

Directions:

Preparing the ingredients.

Melt the coconut oil in a large pot over medium-high heat. Add the onion and cook until soft, about 5 minutes, then add the peas and the water. Bring to a boil, then lower the heat and add the watercress, mint, salt, and pepper.

Cover and simmer for 5 minutes. Stir in the coconut milk, and purée the soup until smooth in a blender or with an immersion blender.

Try this soup with any other fresh, leafy green—anything from spinach to collard greens to arugula to swiss chard.

Nutrition: calories: 178; protein: 6g; total fat: 10g; carbohydrates: 18g; fiber: 5g

# Roasted Red Pepper and Butternut Squash Soup

Preparation time: 10 minutes

Cooking time: 45 minutes

Servings: 6

Ingredients:

1 small butternut squash

1 tablespoon olive oil

1 teaspoon sea salt

2 red bell peppers

1 yellow onion

1 head garlic

2 cups water, or vegetable broth

Zest and juice of 1 lime

1 to 2 tablespoons tahini

Pinch cayenne pepper

½ teaspoon ground coriander

½ teaspoon ground cumin

Toasted squash seeds (optional)

Directions:

Preparing the ingredients.

Preheat the oven to 350°f.

Prepare the squash for roasting by cutting it in half lengthwise, scooping out the seeds, and poking some holes in the flesh with a fork. Reserve the seeds if desired.

Rub a small amount of oil over the flesh and skin, then rub with a bit of sea salt and put the halves skin-side down in a large baking dish. Put it in the oven while you prepare the rest of the vegetables.

Prepare the peppers the exact same way, except they do not need to be poked.

Slice the onion in half and rub oil on the exposed faces. Slice the top off the head of garlic and rub oil on the exposed flesh. After the squash has cooked for 20 minutes, add the peppers, onion, and garlic, and roast for another 20 minutes.

Optionally, you can toast the squash seeds by putting them in the oven in a separate baking dish 10 to 15 minutes before the vegetables are finished.

Keep a close eye on them. When the vegetables are cooked, take them out and let them cool before handling them. The squash will be very soft when poked with a fork.

Scoop the flesh out of the squash skin into a large pot (if you have an immersion blender) or into a blender.

Chop the pepper roughly, remove the onion skin and chop the onion roughly, and squeeze the garlic cloves out of the head, all into the pot or blender. Add the water, the lime zest and juice, and the tahini. Purée the soup, adding more water if you like, to your desired consistency. Season with the salt, cayenne, coriander, and cumin. Serve garnished with toasted squash seeds (if using).

Nutrition: calories: 156; protein: 4g; total fat: 7g; saturated fat: 11g; carbohydrates: 22g; fiber: 5g

# Spinach Soup with Dill and Basil

Preparation time: 10 minutes

Cooking time: 25 minutes

Servings: 8

Ingredients:

1 pound peeled and diced potatoes

1 tablespoon minced garlic

1 teaspoon dry mustard

6 cups vegetable broth

20 ounces chopped frozen spinach

2 cups chopped onion

1 ½ tablespoons salt

½ cup minced dill

1 cup basil

½ teaspoon ground black pepper

Directions:

Whisk onion, garlic, potatoes, broth, mustard, and salt in a pand cook it over medium flame. When it starts boiling, low down the heat and cover it with the lid and cook for 20 minutes. Add the remaining ingredients in it and blend it and cook it for few more minutes and serve it.

Nutrition: Carbohydrates 12g, protein 13g, fats 1g, calories 165.

# Tomato Pumpkin Soup

Preparation time: 25 minutes Cooking time: 15 minutes
Servings: 4

Ingredients:

2 cups pumpkin, diced

1/2 cup tomato, chopped

1/2 cup onion, chopped

1 1/2 tsp curry powder

1/2 tsp paprika

2 cups vegetable stock

1 tsp olive oil

1/2 tsp garlic, minced

Directions:

In a saucepan, add oil, garlic, and onion and sauté for 3
minutes over medium heat.

Add remaining ingredients into the saucepan and bring to boil.

Reduce heat and cover and simmer for 10 minutes.

Puree the soup using a blender until smooth.

Stir well and serve warm.

Nutrition: calories 70; fat 2.7 g; carbohydrates 13.8 g; sugar
6.3 g; protein 1.9 g; cholesterol 0 mg

# Lunch

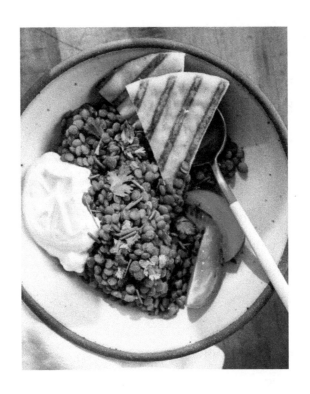

# Vegan Chicken & Rice

Preparation Time: 15 minutes

Cooking Time: 3 hours and 30 minutes

Servings: 8


Ingredients:

8 Tofu thighs

Salt and pepper to taste

½ teaspoon ground coriander

2 teaspoons ground cumin

17 oz. brown rice, cooked

30 oz. black beans

1 tablespoon olive oil

Pinch cayenne pepper

2 cups pico de gallo

¾ cup radish, sliced thinly

2 avocados, sliced


Direction

Season the tofu with salt, pepper, coriander and cumin.

Place in a slow cooker.

Pour in the stock.

Cook on low for 3 hours and 30 minutes.

Place the tofu in a cutting board.

Shred the chicken.

Toss the tofu shreds in the cooking liquid.

Serve the rice in bowls, topped with the tofu and the rest of the ingredients.

Nutrition: Calories: 470 Total fat: 17g Saturated fat: 3g Sodium: 615mg  Carbohydrates: 40g Fiber: 11g Sugar: 1g Protein: 40g

# Eggplant and Olives Stew

Preparation time: 10 minutes

Cooking time: 30 minutes

Servings: 4

Ingredients:

2 scallions, chopped

2 tablespoons avocado oil

2 garlic cloves, chopped

1 bunch parsley, chopped

Salt and black pepper to the taste

1 teaspoon basil, dried

1 teaspoon cumin, dried

2 eggplants, roughly cubed

1 cup green olives, pitted and sliced

3 tablespoons balsamic vinegar

½ Cup tomato passata

Directions:

Heat up a pot with the oil over medium heat, add the scallions, garlic, basil and cumin and sauté for 5 minutes.

Add the eggplants and the other ingredients, toss, cook over medium heat for 25 minutes more, divide into bowls and serve.

Nutrition: calories 93, fat 1.8, fiber 10.6, carbs 18.6, protein 3.4

# Eggplant and Peppers Soup

Preparation time: 10 minutes

Cooking time: 40 minutes

Servings: 4


Ingredients:

2 red bell peppers, chopped

3 scallions, chopped

3 garlic cloves, minced

2 tablespoon olive oil

Salt and black pepper to the taste

5 cups vegetable stock

1 bay leaf

½ cup coconut cream

1 pound eggplants, roughly cubed

2 tablespoons basil, chopped

# Cauliflower and Artichokes Soup

Preparation 10 minutes  Cooking  25 minutes  Servings: 4

Ingredients:

1 pound cauliflower florets

1 cup canned artichoke hearts, drained and chopped

2 scallions, chopped

2 tablespoons olive oil

2 garlic cloves, minced

6 cups vegetable stock

Salt and black pepper to the taste

2/3 cup coconut cream

2 tablespoons cilantro, chopped

Directions:  Heat up a pot with the oil over medium heat, add the scallions and the garlic and sauté for 5 minutes.  Add the cauliflower and the other ingredients, toss, bring to a simmer and cook over medium heat for 20 minutes more.

Blend the soup using an immersion blender, divide it into bowls and serve.

Nutrition: calories 207, fat 17.2, fiber 6.2, carbs 14.1, protein 4.7

Directions:

Heat up a pot with the oil over medium heat, add the scallions and the garlic and sauté for 5 minutes.

Add the peppers and the eggplants and sauté for 5 minutes more.

Add the remaining ingredients, toss, bring to a simmer, cook for 30 minutes, ladle into bowls and serve for lunch.

Nutrition: calories 180, fat 2, fiber 3, carbs 5, protein 10

# Green Pea Fritters

Preparation Time: 10 minutes

Cooking Time: 25 minutes

Serving: 4

Ingredients:

For the Fritters:

1 ½ cups (140 grams) chickpea flour

2 cups (250 grams) frozen peas

1 large white onion, peeled, diced

1 tablespoon minced garlic

1/8 teaspoon salt

1 teaspoon baking soda

2 tablespoons mixed dried Italian herbs

1 tablespoon olive oil

Water as needed

For the Yoghurt Sauce:

1/2 teaspoon dried rosemary

1/2 teaspoon dried parsley

1/2 teaspoon dried mint

1 lemon, juiced

1 cup soy yogurt

Directions:

Switch on the oven, set it to 350° F and let it preheat.

Take a medium saucepan, place it over medium heat, add peas, cover them with water, bring it to a boil, cook for 2 to 3 minutes until tender, and when done, drain the peas and set aside until required.

Take a frying pan, place it over medium heat, add oil and when hot, add onion and garlic; cook for 5 minutes until softened.

Transfer onion-garlic mixture to a food processor, add peas and pulse for 1 minute until the thick paste comes together.

Tip the mixture in a bowl, add salt, baking soda, Italian herbs, and chickpea flour, stir until incorporated and shape the mixture into ten patties.

Brush the patties with oil, arrange them onto a baking sheet and bake for 15 to 18 minutes until golden brown and thoroughly cooked, turning halfway.

Meanwhile, prepare the yogurt sauce: take a medium bowl, add all the ingredients for it and whisk until combined.

Serve fritters with prepared yogurt sauce.

Nutrition: 94 Cal; 2 g Fat; 0 g Saturated Fat; 14 g Carbs; 3 g Fiber; 4 g Protein; 2 g Sugar

# Whipped Potatoes

Preparation Time: 20 minutes

Cooking Time: 35 minutes

Servings: 10


Ingredients:

4 cups water

3 lb. potatoes, sliced into cubes

3 cloves garlic, crushed

6 tablespoons vegan butter

2 bay leaves

10 sage leaves

½ cup Vegan yogurt

¼ cup low-fat milk

Salt to taste


Direction

Boil the potatoes in water for 30 minutes or until tender. Drain.

In a pan over medium heat, cook the garlic in butter for 1 minute.

Add the sage and cook for 5 more minutes.

Discard the garlic.

Use a fork to mash the potatoes.

Whip using an electric mixer while gradually adding the
butter, yogurt, and milk.

Season with salt.

Nutrition: Calories: 169 Total fat: 7.6g Saturated fat: 4.7g
Cholesterol: 21mg Sodium: 251mg Potassium: 519mg
Carbohydrates: 22.1g Fiber: 1.5g  Sugar: 2g Protein: 4.2g

# Quinoa Avocado Salad

Preparation Time: 15 minutes

Cooking Time: 4 minutes

Servings: 4


Ingredients:

2 tablespoons balsamic vinegar

¼ cup cream

¼ cup buttermilk

5 tablespoons freshly squeezed lemon juice, divided

1 clove garlic, grated

2 tablespoons shallot, minced

Salt and pepper to taste

2 tablespoons avocado oil, divided

1 ¼ cups quinoa, cooked

2 heads endive, sliced

2 firm pears, sliced thinly

2 avocados, sliced

¼ cup fresh dill, chopped

Direction

Combine the vinegar, cream, milk, 1 tablespoon lemon juice, garlic, shallot, salt and pepper in a bowl.

Pour 1 tablespoon oil into a pan over medium heat.

Heat the quinoa for 4 minutes.

Transfer quinoa to a plate.

Toss the endive and pears in a mixture of remaining oil, remaining lemon juice, salt and pepper.

Transfer to a plate.

Toss the avocado in the reserved dressing.

Add to the plate.

Top with the dill and quinoa.

Nutrition: Calories: 431 Total fat: 28.5g Saturated fat: 8g Cholesterol: 13mg  Sodium: 345mg Potassium: 779mg Carbohydrates: 42.7g Fiber: 6g Sugar: 3g Protein: 6.6g

# Broccoli Rabe

Preparation Time: 15 minutes Cooking Time: 15 minutes

Servings: 8

Ingredients:

2 oranges, sliced in half

1 lb. broccoli rabe

2 tablespoons sesame oil, toasted

Salt and pepper to taste

1 tablespoon sesame seeds, toasted

Direction

Pour the oil into a pan over medium heat.

Add the oranges and cook until caramelized.

Transfer to a plate.

Put the broccoli in the pan and cook for 8 minutes.

Squeeze the oranges to release juice in a bowl.

Stir in the oil, salt and pepper.

Coat the broccoli rabe with the mixture.

Sprinkle seeds on top.

Nutrition: Calories: 59 Total fat: 4.4g  Saturated fat: 0.6g

Sodium: 164mg  Potassium: 160mg Carbohydrates: 4.1g Fiber:

1.6g Sugar: 2g Protein: 2.2g

# Dinner

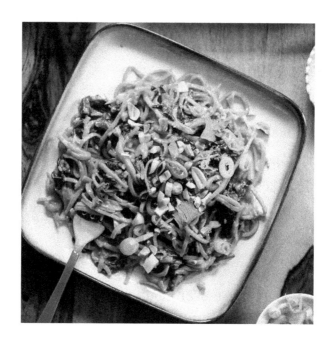

# Green beans stir fry

Preparation time 30 minutes

Cooking time: 10 minutes

Servings: 6-8

Ingredients:

1 1/2 pounds of green beans, stringed, chopped into 1 ½-inch
pieces

1 large onion, thinly sliced

4 star anise (optional)

3 tablespoons avocado oil

1 1/2 tablespoons tamari sauce or soy sauce

Salt to taste

3/4 cup water

Direction: Place a wok over medium heat. Add oil. When oil is
heated, add onions and sauté until onions are translucent.
Add beans, water, tamari sauce, and star anise and stir. Cover
and cook until the beans are tender. Uncover, add salt and
raise the heat to high. Cook until the water dries up in the wok.
Stir a couple of times while cooking.

Collard greens 'n tofu

Preparation time 15 minutes

Cooking time: 20 minutes

Servings: 4

Ingredients:

2 pounds of collard greens, rinsed, chopped

1 cup water

1/2 pound of tofu, chopped

Salt to taste

Pepper powder to taste

Crushed red chili to taste

Direction:

Place a large skillet over medium-high heat. Add oil. When the oil is heated, add tofu and cook until brown.

Add rest of the ingredients and mix well.

Cook until greens wilts and almost dry.

# Broccoli & black beans stir fry

Preparation time 60 minutes

Cooking time: 10 minutes

Servings: 6


Ingredients:

4 cups broccoli flore ts

2 cups cooked black beans

1 tablespoon sesame oil

4 teaspoons sesame seeds

2 cloves garlic, finely minced

2 teaspoons ginger, finely chopped

A large pinch red chili flakes

A pinch turmeric powder

Salt to taste

Lime juice to taste (optional)

Direction:

Steam broccoli for 6 minutes. Drain and set aside.

Warm the sesame oil in a large frying pan over medium heat.

Add sesame seeds, chili flakes, ginger, garlic, turmeric powder, and salt. Sauté for a couple of minutes.

Add broccoli and black beans and sauté until thoroughly heated.

Sprinkle lime juice and serve hot.

# Smoothies, Snacks and Desserts

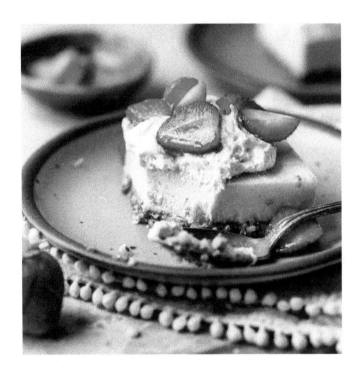

# Warm Pomegranate Punch

Preparation time: 3 hours and 15 minutes

Cooking time: 3 hours

Servings: 10


Ingredients:

3 cinnamon sticks, each about 3 inches long

12 whole cloves

1/2 cup of coconut sugar

1/3 cup of lemon juice

32 fluid ounce of pomegranate juice

32 fluid ounce of apple juice, unsweetened

16 fluid ounce of brewed tea


Directions:

Using a 4-quart slow cooker, pour the lemon juice, pomegranate, juice apple juice, tea, and then sugar.

Wrap the whole cloves and cinnamon stick in a cheese cloth, tie its corners with a string, and immerse it in the liquid present in the slow cooker.

Then cover it with the lid, plug in the slow cooker and let it cook at the low heat setting for 3 hours or until it is heated thoroughly.

When done, discard the cheesecloth bag and serve it hot or cold.

Nutrition:  Calories:253 Cal, Carbohydrates:58g, Protein:7g, Fats:2g, Fiber:3g.

# Raspberry Protein Shake

Preparation Time: 5 min.

Cooking Time: 5 min.

Serving: 1

Ingredients:

¼ avocado

1 c. raspberries, frozen

1 scoop protein powder

½ c. almond milk

Ice cubes

Directions:

In a high-speed blender add all the ingredients and blend until lumps of fruit disappear.

Add two to four ice cubes and blend to your desired consistency.

Serve immediately and enjoy!

Nutrition: Calories: 756 | Carbohydrates: 80.1 g | Proteins: 27.6 g | Fats: 40.7 g

# Nice Spiced Cherry Cider

Preparation time: 4 hours and 5 minutes

Cooking time: 4 hours

Servings: 16

Ingredients:

2 cinnamon sticks, each about 3 inches long

6-ounce of cherry gelatin

4 quarts of apple cider

Directions:

Using a 6-quarts slow cooker, pour the apple cider and add the cinnamon stick.

Stir, then cover the slow cooker with its lid. Plug in the cooker and let it cook for 3 hours at the high heat setting or until it is heated thoroughly.

Then add and stir the gelatin properly, then continue cooking for another hour.

When done, remove the cinnamon sticks and serve the drink hot or cold.

Nutrition: , Calories:100 Cal, Carbohydrates:0g, Protein:0g, Fats:0g, Fiber:0g.

# Fruity Smoothie

Preparation Time: 10 Minutes Cooking time: 0 minute

Servings: 1

Ingredients:

¾ cup soy yogurt

½ cup pineapple juice

1 cup pineapple chunks

1 cup raspberries, sliced

1 cup blueberries, sliced

Direction:

Process the ingredients in a blender. Chill before serving.

Nutrition: Calories 279, Total Fat 2 g, Saturated Fat 0 g

Cholesterol 4 mg, Sodium 149 mg, Total Carbohydrate 56 g

Dietary Fiber 7 g, Protein 12 g, Total Sugars 46 g  Potassium

719 mg

# Strawberry Cupcakes With Cashew Cheese Frosting

Preparation Time: 35 minutes + 30 minutes chilling

Servings: 4

To make this lovely pink ganache, you just need three basic ingredients. With freshly strawberry puree, it takes on a buttery flavor.

Ingredients

For the cupcakes:

2 cups whole-wheat flour

¼ cup cornstarch

2 ½ tsp baking powder

1 ½ cups pure date sugar

½ tsp salt

¾ cup unsalted plant butter, room temperature

3 tsp vanilla extract

1 cup strawberries, pureed

1 cup oat milk, room temperature

For the frosting:

¾ cup cashew cream

2 tbsp coconut oil, melted

3 tbsp pure maple syrup

1 tsp vanilla extract

1 tsp freshly squeezed lemon juice

¼ tsp salt

2-4 tbsp water as needed for blending

Directions

Preheat the oven to 350 F and line a 12-holed muffin tray with cupcake liners. Set aside.

In a large bowl, mix the flour, cornstarch, baking powder, date sugar, and salt.

Using an electric mixer, whisk in the plant butter, vanilla extract, strawberries, and oat milk until well combined.

Divide the mixture into the muffin cups two-thirds way up and bake in the oven for 20 to 25 minutes or until golden brown on top and a toothpick inserted comes out clean. Remove the cupcakes and allow cooling while you make the frosting.

In a blender, add the cashew cream, coconut oil, maple syrup, vanilla, lemon juice, and salt. Process until smooth. If the mixture is too thick, add some water to lighten the consistency a little. Pour the frosting into medium and chill for 30 minutes.

Transfer the mixture into a piping bag and swirl mounds of the frosting onto the cupcakes. Serve immediately.

Nutritional info per serving

Calories 853 | Fats 42g| Carbs 112.8g | Protein 14.3g

# Summer Banana Pudding

Preparation Time: 25 minutes + 1 hour

Servings: 4

It's a no bake dessert that's perfect for a group's last minute get together. Just that something that everyone loves!

Ingredients

1 cup unsweetened almond milk

2 cups cashew cream

¾ cup + 1 tbsp pure date sugar

¼ tsp salt

3 tbsp cornstarch

2 tbsp cold plant butter, cut into 4 pieces

1 tsp vanilla extract

2 medium banana, peeled and sliced

Directions

In a medium pot, mix the almond milk, cashew cream, date sugar, and salt. Cook over medium heat until slightly thickened, 10 to 15 minutes.

Stir in the cornstarch, plant butter, vanilla extract, and banana extract. Cook further for 1 to 2 minutes or until the pudding thickens. Dish the pudding into 4 serving bowls and chill in the refrigerator for at least 1 hour. To serve, top with the bananas and enjoy!

Nutritional info per serving

Calories 466 | Fats 29.9g| Carbs 47.8g | Protein 4.3g

# Energizing Ginger Detox Tonic

Preparation time: 15 minutes

Cooking time: 10 minutes

Servings: 2

Ingredients:

1/2 teaspoon of grated ginger, fresh

1 small lemon slice

1/8 teaspoon of cayenne pepper

1/8 teaspoon of ground turmeric

1/8 teaspoon of ground cinnamon

1 teaspoon of maple syrup

1 teaspoon of apple cider vinegar

2 cups of boiling water

Directions:

Pour the boiling water into a small saucepan, add and stir the ginger, then let it rest for 8 to 10 minutes, before covering the pan.

Pass the mixture through a strainer and into the liquid, add the cayenne pepper, turmeric, cinnamon and stir properly.

Add the maple syrup, vinegar, and lemon slice.

Add and stir an infused lemon and serve immediately.

Nutrition: Calories:80 Cal, Carbohydrates:0g, Protein:0g, Fats:0g, Fiber:0g.

# Fragrant Spiced Coffee

Preparation time: 3 hours and 10 minutes

Cooking time: 3 hours

Servings: 8


Ingredients:

4 cinnamon sticks, each about 3 inches long

1 1/2 teaspoons of whole cloves

1/3 cup of honey

2-ounce of chocolate syrup

1/2 teaspoon of anise extract

8 cups of brewed coffee


Directions:

Pour the coffee in a 4-quarts slow cooker and pour in the remaining ingredients except for cinnamon and stir properly. Wrap the whole cloves in cheesecloth and tie its corners with strings.

Immerse this cheesecloth bag in the liquid present in the slow cooker and cover it with the lid.

Then plug in the slow cooker and let it cook on the low heat setting for 3 hours or until heated thoroughly.

When done, discard the cheesecloth bag and serve.

Nutrition: Calories:150 Cal, Carbohydrates:35g, Protein:3g, Fats:0g, Fiber:0g.

# Warm Spiced Lemon Drink

Preparation time: 2 hours and 10 minutes

Cooking time: 2 hours

Servings: 12

Ingredients:

1 cinnamon stick, about 3 inches long

1/2 teaspoon of whole cloves

2 cups of coconut sugar

4 fluid of ounce pineapple juice

1/2 cup and 2 tablespoons of lemon juice

12 fluid ounce of orange juice

2 1/2 quarts of water

Directions:

Pour water into a 6-quarts slow cooker and stir the sugar and lemon juice properly.

Wrap the cinnamon, the whole cloves in cheesecloth and tie its corners with string. Immerse this cheesecloth bag in the liquid present in the slow cooker and cover it with the lid.

Then plug in the slow cooker and let it cook on high heat setting for 2 hours or until it is heated thoroughly.

When done, discard the cheesecloth bag and serve the drink hot or cold.

Nutrition: Calories:15 Cal, Carbohydrates:3.2g, Protein:0.1g, Fats:0g, Fiber:0g.

# Apple Raspberry Cobbler

Preparation Time: 50 minutes

Servings: 4

A safer type of fruit cobbler where a cut in sugar enhances the fruit.

Ingredients

3 apples, peeled, cored, and chopped

2 tbsp pure date sugar

1 cup fresh raspberries

2 tbsp unsalted plant butter

½ cup whole-wheat flour

1 cup toasted rolled oats

2 tbsp pure date sugar

1 tsp cinnamon powder

Directions

Preheat the oven to 350 F and grease a baking dish with some plant butter.

Add the apples, date sugar, and 3 tbsp of water to a medium pot. Cook over low heat until the date sugar melts and then, mix in the raspberries. Cook until the fruits soften, 10 minutes. Pour and spread the fruit mixture into the baking dish and set aside.

In a blender, add the plant butter, flour, oats, date sugar, and cinnamon powder. Pulse a few times until crumbly.

Spoon and spread the mixture on the fruit mix until evenly layered.

Bake in the oven for 25 to 30 minutes or until golden brown on top.

Remove the dessert, allow cooling for 2 minutes, and serve.

Nutritional info per serving

Calories 539 | Fats 12g| Carbs 105.7g | Protein 8.2g

# White Chocolate Pudding

Preparation Time: 4 hours 20 minutes

Servings: 4


Ingredients

3 tbsp flax seed + 9 tbsp water

3 tbsp cornstarch

¼ tbsp salt

1 cup cashew cream

2 ½ cups almond milk

½ pure date sugar

1 tbsp vanilla caviar

6 oz unsweetened white chocolate chips

Whipped coconut cream for topping

Sliced bananas and raspberries for topping


Directions

In a small bowl, mix the flax seed powder with water and allow thickening for 5 minutes to make the flax egg.

In a large bowl, whisk the cornstarch and salt, and then slowly mix in the in the cashew cream until smooth. Whisk in the flax egg until well combined.

Pour the almond milk into a pot and whisk in the date sugar. Cook over medium heat while frequently stirring until the sugar dissolves. Reduce the heat to low and simmer until steamy and bubbly around the edges.

Pour half of the almond milk mixture into the flax egg mix, whisk well and pour this mixture into the remaining milk content in the pot. Whisk continuously until well combined. Bring the new mixture to a boil over medium heat while still frequently stirring and scraping all the corners of the pot, 2 minutes.

Turn the heat off, stir in the vanilla caviar, then the white chocolate chips until melted. Spoon the mixture into a bowl, allow cooling for 2 minutes, cover with plastic wraps making sure to press the plastic onto the surface of the pudding, and refrigerate for 4 hours.

Remove the pudding from the fridge, take off the plastic wrap and whip for about a minute.

Spoon the dessert into serving cups, swirl some coconut whipping cream on top, and top with the bananas and raspberries. Enjoy immediately.

Nutritional info per serving

Calories 654 | Fats 47.9g| Carbs 52.1g | Protein 7.3g

# All Purpose Dill Seed Rub

Boost your steak with vibrant, spiced flavors of this all-purpose dill seed rub. It also beautifully seasons chicken and pork meat cuts. Apply this unique rub minutes before grilling or cooking; you can also store it at room temperature for 12-14 days without sacrificing on its quality.

Preparation Time: 5 min.

Cooking Time: 5 min.

Servings: 6-7 tsp.

Ingredients:

Paprika - 2 tsp.

Ground coriander - 2 tsp.

Dill seed – 1 tsp.

Dry mustard - ½ tsp.

Garlic, minced – 1 clove

Black pepper and salt as required

Cayenne pepper - ¼ tsp.

Directions:

Mix in all the rub ingredients in your mixing bowl to make the dill seed rub. Gently mix all ingredients using spatula or spoon to form an aromatic rub mixture.

Now, take your choice of meat cut and place it on a firm surface. Brush the freshly made rub on it; pat gently for the rub to stick onto the surface. Turn the meat cut and repeat to spice up its other side. Repeat with other meat cuts.

Let your meat cuts adequately season for more rich flavors for a few hours in your refrigerator. Take them out, as they are ready to be cooked or grilled!

# Classic Pecan Pie

Preparation Time: 50 minutes + 1 hour chilling

Servings: 4

The traditional pie is baked to a lustrous brown pecan load.

Ingredients

For the piecrust:

4 tbsp flax seed powder + 12 tbsp water

1/3 cup whole-wheat flour + more for dusting

½ tsp salt

¼ cup plant butter, cold and crumbled

3 tbsp pure malt syrup

1 ½ tsp vanilla extract.

For the filling:

3 tbsp flax seed powder + 9 tbsp water

2 cups toasted pecans, coarsely chopped

1 cup light corn syrup

½ cup pure date sugar

1 tbsp pure pomegranate molasses

4 tbsp plant butter, melted

½ tsp salt

2 tsp vanilla extract

Directions

Preheat the oven to 350 F and grease a large pie pan with cooking spray.

In a medium bowl, mix the flax seed powder with water and allow thickening for 5 minutes. Do this for the filling's flax egg too in a separate bowl.

In a large bowl, combine the flour and salt. Add the plant butter and using an electric hand mixer, whisk until crumbly. Pour in the crust's flax egg, maple syrup, vanilla, and mix until smooth dough forms.

Flatten the dough on a flat surface, cover with plastic wrap, and refrigerate for 1 hour.

After, lightly dust a working surface with flour, remove the dough onto the surface, and using a rolling pin, flatten the dough into a 1-inch diameter circle.

Lay the dough on the pie pan and press to fit the shape of the pan. Use a knife to trim the edges of the pan. Lay a parchment paper on the dough, pour on some baking beans and bake in the oven until golden brown, 15 to 20 minutes. Remove the pan from the oven, pour out the baking beans, and allow cooling.

In a large bowl, mix the filling's flax egg, pecans, corn syrup, date sugar, pomegranate molasses, plant butter, salt, and vanilla. Pour and spread the mixture on the piecrust. Bake further for 20 minutes or until the filling sets. Remove from the oven, decorate with more pecans, slice, and cool. Slice and serve.

Nutritional info per serving

Calories 992 | Fats 59.8g| Carbs 117.6 g | Protein 8g

# Tangy Spiced Cranberry Drink

Preparation time: 3 hours and 10 minutes

Cooking time: 3 hours

Servings: 14

Ingredients:

1 1/2 cups of coconut sugar

12 whole cloves

2 fluid ounce of lemon juice

6 fluid ounce of orange juice

32 fluid ounce of cranberry juice

8 cups of hot water

1/2 cup of Red Hot candies

Directions:

Pour the water into a 6-quarts slow cooker along with the cranberry juice, orange juice, and the lemon juice.

Stir the sugar properly. Wrap the whole cloves in a cheese cloth, tie its corners with strings, and immerse it in the liquid present inside the slow cooker. Add the red hot candies to the slow cooker and cover it with the lid. Then plug in the slow cooker and let it cook on the low heat setting for 3 hours or until it is heated thoroughly.

When done, discard the cheesecloth bag and serve.

Nutrition: Calories:89 Cal, Carbohydrates:27g, Protein:0g, Fats:0g, Fiber:1g.

# Soothing Ginger Tea Drink

Preparation time: 2 hours and 15 minutes

Cooking time: 2 hours and 10 minutes

Servings: 8


Ingredients:

1 tablespoon of minced ginger root

2 tablespoons of honey

15 green tea bags

32 fluid ounce of white grape juice

2 quarts of boiling water


Directions:

Pour water into a 4-quarts slow cooker, immerse tea bags, cover the cooker and let stand for 10 minutes.

After 10 minutes, remove and discard tea bags and stir in remaining ingredients.

Return cover to slow cooker, then plug in and let cook at high heat setting for 2 hours or until heated through.

When done, strain the liquid and serve hot or cold.

Nutrition: Calories:45 Cal, Carbohydrates:12g, Protein:0g, Fats:0g, Fiber:0g.

# Chocolate & Pistachio Popsicles

Preparation Time: 5 minutes + 3 hours chilling

Servings: 4

A popsicle is one of those wonders full of endless possibilities that are creative and mouth-watering.

Ingredients

½ cup unsweetened chocolate chips, melted

1 ½ cups oat milk

1 tbsp unsweetened cocoa powder

3 tbsp pure date syrup

1 tsp vanilla extract

A handful pistachios, chopped

Directions  In a blender, add chocolate, oat milk, cocoa powder, date syrup, vanilla, pistachios, and process until smooth. Divide the mixture into popsicle molds and freeze for 3 hours. Dip the popsicle molds in warm water to loosen the popsicles and pull out the popsicles.

Nutritional info per serving

Calories 315 | Fats 17.8g| Carbs 34.9g | Protein 11.9g

# Nut Stuffed Sweet Apples

Preparation Time: 35 minutes

Servings: 4

This nut Stuffed Baked Apples are a buzz-friendly sliding dessert, or say, one or two weekend desserts snack.

Ingredients

4 gala apples

3 tbsp pure maple syrup

4 tbsp almond flour

6 tbsp pure date sugar

6 tbsp plant butter, cold and cued

1 cup chopped mixed nuts

Directions

Preheat the oven the 400 F.

Slice off the top of the apples and use a melon baller or spoon to scoop out the cores of the apples. In a bowl, mix the maple syrup, almond flour, date sugar, butter, and nuts.

Spoon the mixture into the apples and then bake in the oven for 25 minutes or until the nuts are golden brown on top and the apples soft. Remove the apples from the oven, allow cooling, and serve.

Nutritional info per serving

Calories 581 | Fats 43.6g| Carbs 52.1g | Protein 3.6g

# Vanilla Milkshake

Preparation Time: 5 min.

Cooking Time: 5 min.

Servings: 4


Ingredients:

2 c. ice cubes

2 t. vanilla extract

6 tbsp. powdered erythritol

1 c. cream of dairy-free

½ c. coconut milk


Directions:

In a high-speed blender, add all the ingredients and blend.

Add ice cubes and blend until smooth.

Serve immediately and enjoy!

Nutrition: Calories: 125 | Carbohydrates: 6.8 g | Proteins: 1.2 g | Fats: 11.5 g

# Raspberry Almond Smoothie

Preparation Time: 5 min.

Cooking Time: 5 min.

Serving: 1


Ingredients:

10 Almonds, finely chopped

3 tbsp. almond butter

1 c. almond milk

1 c. Raspberries, frozen


Directions:

In a high-speed blender, add all the ingredients and blend until smooth.

Serve immediately and enjoy!

Nutrition: Calories: 449 | Carbohydrates: 26 g | Proteins: 14 g | Fats: 35 g

# Sauce Recipes

## Vegan High-Protein Queso

Preparation time: 5 minutes

Cooking time: 5 minutes

Servings: 2

Ingredients:

1/4 cup nutritional yeast

1/2 block tofu

3 tablespoon lemon juice

1/4 teaspoon tapioca starch

1/4 teaspoon garlic powder

1/4 teaspoon turmeric

1/4 teaspoon onion powder

1/4 cup water

1/2 teaspoon salt

Directions:

Add tofu, yeast, starch, lemon juice, salt, garlic powder, turmeric and onion powder and blend until well mixed. Add water as desired. Heat in a microwave for 30 seconds. Serve and enjoy.

# Tahini Maple Dressing

Preparation time: 5 minutes

Cooking time: 5 minutes

Servings: 4 oz

Ingredients

¼ cup tahini

1 ½ tablespoons maple syrup

2 teaspoons lemon juice

¼ cup of water

1/8 teaspoon Himalayan pink salt

Directions:

Add all the ingredients to a bowl, Stir well to combine, until well mixed.

Use as a dressing for the salad or other dishes. Store in a fridge.

# Meal Plans

## Meal Plan 1

| Day | Breakfast | Lunch | Dinner | Snacks |
|---|---|---|---|---|
| 1 | Chocolate PB Smoothie | Cauliflower Latke | Noodles Alfredo with Herby Tofu | Beans with Sesame Hummus |
| 2 | Orange french toast | Roasted Brussels Sprouts | Lemon Couscous with Tempeh Kabobs | Candied Honey-Coconut Peanuts |
| 3 | Oatmeal Raisin Breakfast Cookie | Brussels Sprouts & Cranberries Salad | Portobello Burger with Veggie Fries | Choco Walnuts Fat Bombs |
| 4 | Berry Beetsicle Smoothie | Potato Latke | Thai Seitan Vegetable Curry | Crispy Honey Pecans (Slow Cooker) |
| 5 | Blueberry Oat Muffins | Broccoli Rabe | Tofu Cabbage Stir-Fry | Crunchy Fried Pickles |

| | | | |
|---|---|---|---|
| 6 | Quinoa Applesauce Muffins | Whipped Potatoes | Curried Tofu with Buttery Cabbage | Granola bars with Maple Syrup |
| 7 | Pumpkin pancakes | Quinoa Avocado Salad | Smoked Tempeh with Broccoli Fritters | Green Soy Beans Hummus |
| 8 | Green breakfast smoothie | Roasted Sweet Potatoes | Cheesy Potato Casserole | High Protein Avocado Guacamole |
| 9 | Blueberry Lemonade Smoothie | Cauliflower Salad | Curry Mushroom Pie | Homemade Energy Nut Bars |
| 10 | Berry Protein Smoothie | Garlic Mashed Potatoes & Turnips | Spicy Cheesy Tofu Balls | Honey Peanut Butter |
| 11 | Blueberry and chia smoothie | Green Beans with Bacon | Radish Chips | Mediterranean Marinated Olives |
| 12 | Green Kickstart Smoothie | Coconut Brussels Sprouts | Sautéed Pears | Nut Butter & Dates Granola |

| | | | | |
|---|---|---|---|---|
| 13 | Warm Maple and Cinnamon Quinoa | Cod Stew with Rice & Sweet Potatoes | Pecan & Blueberry Crumble | Oven-baked Caramelize Plantains |
| 14 | Warm Quinoa Breakfast Bowl | Chicken & Rice | Rice Pudding | Powerful Peas & Lentils Dip |
| 15 | Banana Bread Rice Pudding | Rice Bowl with Edamame | Mango Sticky Rice | Protein "Raffaello" Candies |
| 16 | Apple and cinnamon oatmeal | Chickpea Avocado Sandwich | Noodles Alfredo with Herby Tofu | Protein-Rich Pumpkin Bowl |
| 17 | Mango Key Lime Pie Smoothie | Roasted Tomato Sandwich | Lemon Couscous with Tempeh Kabobs | Savory Red Potato-Garlic Balls |
| 18 | Spiced orange breakfast couscous | Pulled "Pork" Sandwiches | Portobello Burger with Veggie Fries | Spicy Smooth Red Lentil Dip |

| 19 | Breakfast parfaits | Cauliflower Latke | Thai Seitan Vegetable Curry | Steamed Broccoli with Sesame |
|---|---|---|---|---|
| 20 | Sweet potato and kale hash | Roasted Brussels Sprouts | Tofu Cabbage Stir-Fry | Vegan Eggplant Patties |
| 21 | Delicious Oat Meal | Brussels Sprouts & Cranberries Salad | Curried Tofu with Buttery Cabbage | Vegan Breakfast Sandwich |
| 22 | Breakfast Cherry Delight | Potato Latke | Smoked Tempeh with Broccoli Fritters | Chickpea And Mushroom Burger |
| 23 | Crazy Maple and Pear Breakfast | Broccoli Rabe | Cheesy Potato Casserole | Beans with Sesame Hummus |
| 24 | Hearty French Toast Bowls | Whipped Potatoes | Curry Mushroom Pie | Candied Honey-Coconut Peanuts |
| 25 | Chocolate PB Smoothie | Quinoa Avocado Salad | Spicy Cheesy Tofu Balls | Choco Walnuts Fat Bombs |

| 26 | Orange french toast | Roasted Sweet Potatoes | Radish Chips | Crispy Honey Pecans (Slow Cooker) |
|----|---------------------|------------------------|-------------|-----------------------------------|
| 27 | Oatmeal Raisin Breakfast Cookie | Cauliflower Salad | Sautéed Pears | Crunchy Fried Pickles |
| 28 | Berry Beetsicle Smoothie | Garlic Mashed Potatoes & Turnips | Pecan & Blueberry Crumble | Granola bars with Maple Syrup |

# Meal Plan 2

| Day | Breakfast | Lunch | Dinner | Smoothie |
|-----|-----------|-------|--------|----------|
| 1 | Mexican-Spiced Tofu Scramble | Teriyaki Tofu Stir-fry | Mushroom Steak | Chocolate Smoothie |
| 2 | Whole Grain Protein Bowl | Red Lentil and Quinoa Fritters | Spicy Grilled Tofu Steak | Chocolate Mint Smoothie |
| 3 | Healthy Breakfast Bowl | Green Pea Fritters | Piquillo Salsa Verde Steak | Cinnamon Roll Smoothie |
| 4 | Healthy Breakfast Bowl | Breaded Tofu Steaks | Butternut Squash Steak | Coconut Smoothie |
| 5 | Root Vegetable Hash With Avocado Crème | Chickpea and Edamame Salad | Cauliflower Steak Kicking Corn | Maca Almond Smoothie |
| 6 | Chocolate Strawberry Almond Protein Smoothie | Thai Tofu and Quinoa Bowls | Pistachio Watermelon Steak | Blueberry Smoothie |

| 7 | Banana Bread Breakfast Muffins | Black Bean and Bulgur Chili | BBQ Ribs | Nutty Protein Shake |
|---|---|---|---|---|
| 8 | Stracciatella Muffins | Cauliflower Steaks | Spicy Veggie Steaks With veggies | Cinnamon Pear Smoothie |
| 9 | Cardamom Persimmon Scones With Maple-Persimmon Cream | Avocado and Hummus Sandwich | Mushroom Steak | Vanilla Milkshake |
| 10 | Activated Buckwheat & Coconut Porridge With Blueberry Sauce | Chickpea Spinach Salad | Spicy Grilled Tofu Steak | Raspberry Protein Shake |
| 11 | Sweet Molasses Brown Bread | Teriyaki Tofu Stir-fry | Piquillo Salsa Verde Steak | Raspberry Almond Smoothie |
| 12 | Mexican-Spiced Tofu Scramble | Red Lentil and Quinoa Fritters | Butternut Squash Steak | Chocolate Smoothie |

| 13 | Whole Grain Protein Bowl | Green Pea Fritters | Cauliflower Steak Kicking Corn | Chocolate Mint Smoothie |
|---|---|---|---|---|
| 14 | Healthy Breakfast Bowl | Breaded Tofu Steaks | Pistachio Watermelon Steak | Cinnamon Roll Smoothie |
| 15 | Healthy Breakfast Bowl | Chickpea and Edamame Salad | BBQ Ribs | Coconut Smoothie |
| 16 | Root Vegetable Hash With Avocado Crème | Thai Tofu and Quinoa Bowls | Spicy Veggie Steaks With veggies | Maca Almond Smoothie |
| 17 | Chocolate Strawberry Almond Protein Smoothie | Black Bean and Bulgur Chili | Mushroom Steak | Blueberry Smoothie |
| 18 | Banana Bread Breakfast Muffins | Cauliflower Steaks | Spicy Grilled Tofu Steak | Nutty Protein Shake |
| 19 | Stracciatella Muffins | Avocado and Hummus Sandwich | Piquillo Salsa Verde Steak | Cinnamon Pear Smoothie |

| 20 | Cardamom Persimmon Scones With Maple-Persimmon Cream | Chickpea Spinach Salad | Butternut Squash Steak | Vanilla Milkshake |
|----|----|----|----|----|
| 21 | Activated Buckwheat & Coconut Porridge With Blueberry Sauce | Teriyaki Tofu Stir-fry | Cauliflower Steak Kicking Corn | Raspberry Protein Shake |
| 22 | Sweet Molasses Brown Bread | Red Lentil and Quinoa Fritters | Pistachio Watermelon Steak | Raspberry Almond Smoothie |
| 23 | Mexican-Spiced Tofu Scramble | Green Pea Fritters | BBQ Ribs | Chocolate Smoothie |
| 24 | Whole Grain Protein Bowl | Breaded Tofu Steaks | Spicy Veggie Steaks With veggies | Chocolate Mint Smoothie |
| 25 | Healthy Breakfast Bowl | Chickpea and Edamame Salad | Mushroom Steak | Cinnamon Roll Smoothie |

| 26 | Healthy Breakfast Bowl | Thai Tofu and Quinoa Bowls | Spicy Grilled Tofu Steak | Coconut Smoothie |
|----|------------------------|----------------------------|--------------------------|------------------|
| 27 | Root Vegetable Hash With Avocado Crème | Black Bean and Bulgur Chili | Piquillo Salsa Verde Steak | Maca Almond Smoothie |
| 28 | Chocolate Strawberry Almond Protein Smoothie | Cauliflower Steaks | Butternut Squash Steak | Blueberry Smoothie |

# Meal Plan 3

| Day | Breakfast | Lunch | Dinner | Snacks |
|-----|-----------|-------|--------|--------|
| 1 | Breakfast Blueberry Muffins | Quinoa Buddha Bowl | Broccoli & black beans stir fry | Spiced Chickpeas |
| 2 | Oatmeal with Pears | Lettuce Hummus Wrap | Stuffed peppers | Lemon & Ginger Kale Chips |
| 3 | Yogurt with Cucumber | Simple Curried Vegetable Rice | Sweet 'n spicy tofu | Chocolate Energy Snack Bar |
| 4 | Breakfast Casserole | Spicy Southwestern Hummus Wraps | Eggplant & mushrooms in peanut sauce | Hazelnut & Maple Chia Crunch |
| 5 | Berries with Mascarpone on Toasted Bread | Buffalo Cauliflower Wings | Green beans stir fry | Roasted Cauliflower |
| 6 | Fruit Cup | Veggie Fritters | Collard greens 'n tofu | Apple Cinnamon Crisps |
| 7 | Oatmeal with Black Beans & Cheddar | Pizza Bites | Cassoulet | Pumpkin Spice Granola Bites |

| 8 | Breakfast Smoothie | Avocado, Spinach and Kale Soup | Double-garlic bean and vegetable soup | Salted Carrot Fries |
|---|---|---|---|---|
| 9 | Yogurt with Beets & Raspberries | Curry spinach soup | Mean bean minestrone | Zesty Orange Muffins |
| 10 | Curry Oatmeal | Arugula and Artichokes Bowls | Grilled Halloumi Broccoli Salad | Chocolate Tahini Balls |
| 11 | Fig & Cheese Oatmeal | Minty arugula soup | Black Bean Lentil Salad With Lime Dressing | Spiced Chickpeas |
| 12 | Pumpkin Oats | Spinach and Broccoli Soup | Arugula Lentil Salad | Lemon & Ginger Kale Chips |
| 13 | Sweet Potato Toasts | Coconut zucchini cream | Red Cabbage Salad With Curried Seitan | Chocolate Energy Snack Bar |
| 14 | Tofu Scramble Tacos | Zucchini and Cauliflower Soup | Chickpea, Red Kidney Bean And Feta Salad | Hazelnut & Maple Chia Crunch |

| 15 | Almond Chia Pudding | Chard soup | The Amazing Chickpea Spinach Salad | Roasted Cauliflower |
|---|---|---|---|---|
| 16 | Breakfast Parfait Popsicles | Avocado, Pine Nuts and Chard Salad | Curried Carrot Slaw With Tempeh | Apple Cinnamon Crisps |
| 17 | Strawberry Smoothie Bowl | Grapes, Avocado and Spinach Salad | Black & White Bean Quinoa Salad | Pumpkin Spice Granola Bites |
| 18 | Peanut Butter Granola | Greens and Olives Pan | Greek Salad With Seitan Gyros Strips | Salted Carrot Fries |
| 19 | Apple Chia Pudding | Mushrooms and Chard Soup | Chickpea And Edamame Salad | Zesty Orange Muffins |
| 20 | Pumpkin Spice Bites | Tomato, Green Beans and Chard Soup | Broccoli & black beans stir fry | Chocolate Tahini Balls |
| 21 | Lemon Spelt Scones | Hot roasted peppers cream | Stuffed peppers | Spiced Chickpeas |
| 22 | Veggie Breakfast Scramble | Eggplant and Peppers Soup | Sweet 'n spicy tofu | Lemon & Ginger Kale Chips |

| 23 | Breakfast Blueberry Muffins | Eggplant and Olives Stew | Eggplant & mushrooms in peanut sauce | Chocolate Energy Snack Bar |
|---|---|---|---|---|
| 24 | Oatmeal with Pears | Cauliflower and Artichokes Soup | Green beans stir fry | Hazelnut & Maple Chia Crunch |
| 25 | Yogurt with Cucumber | Quinoa Buddha Bowl | Collard greens 'n tofu | Roasted Cauliflower |
| 26 | Breakfast Casserole | Lettuce Hummus Wrap | Cassoulet | Apple Cinnamon Crisps |
| 27 | Berries with Mascarpone on Toasted Bread | Simple Curried Vegetable Rice | Double-garlic bean and vegetable soup | Pumpkin Spice Granola Bites |
| 28 | Fruit Cup | Spicy Southwestern Hummus Wraps | Mean bean minestrone | Salted Carrot Fries |

# Meal plan 4

| Day | Breakfast | Entrées | Soup , Salad, & Sides | Smoothie |
|---|---|---|---|---|
| 1 | Tasty Oatmeal Muffins | Black Bean Dip | Spinach Soup with Dill and Basil | Fruity Smoothie |
| 2 | Omelet with Chickpea Flour | Cannellini Bean Cashew Dip | Coconut Watercress Soup | Energizing Ginger Detox Tonic |
| 3 | White Sandwich Bread | Cauliflower Popcorn | Coconut Watercress Soup | Warm Spiced Lemon Drink |
| 4 | A Toast to Remember | Cinnamon Apple Chips with Dip | Coconut Watercress Soup | Soothing Ginger Tea Drink |
| 5 | Tasty Panini | Crunchy Asparagus Spears | Cauliflower Spinach Soup | Nice Spiced Cherry Cider |

| 6 | Tasty Oatmeal and Carrot Cake | Cucumber Bites with Chive and Sunflower Seeds | Avocado Mint Soup | Fragrant Spiced Coffee |
|---|---|---|---|---|
| 7 | Onion & Mushroom Tart with a Nice Brown Rice Crust | Garlicky Kale Chips | Creamy Squash Soup | Tangy Spiced Cranberry Drink |
| 8 | Perfect Breakfast Shake | Hummus-stuffed Baby Potatoes | Cucumber Edamame Salad | Warm Pomegranate Punch |
| 9 | Beet Gazpacho | Homemade Trail Mix | Best Broccoli Salad | Rich Truffle Hot Chocolate |
| 10 | Vegetable Rice | Nut Butter Maple Dip | Rainbow Orzo Salad | Ultimate Mulled Wine |
| 11 | Courgette Risotto | Oven Baked Sesame Fries | Broccoli Pasta Salad | Pleasant Lemonade |
| 12 | Country Breakfast Cereal | Pumpkin Orange Spice Hummus | Eggplant & Roasted Tomato Farro Salad | Pineapple, Banana & Spinach Smoothie |

| 13 | Oatmeal Fruit Shake | Quick English Muffin Mexican Pizzas | Garden Patch Sandwiches on Multigrain Bread | Kale & Avocado Smoothie |
|---|---|---|---|---|
| 14 | Amaranth Banana Breakfast Porridge | Quinoa Trail Mix Cups | Garden Salad Wraps | Coconut & Strawberry Smoothie |
| 15 | Green Ginger Smoothie | Black Bean Dip | Marinated Mushroom Wraps | Pumpkin Chia Smoothie |
| 16 | Orange Dream Creamsicle | Cannellini Bean Cashew Dip | Tamari Toasted Almonds | Cantaloupe Smoothie Bowl |
| 17 | Strawberry Limeade | Cauliflower Popcorn | Nourishing Whole-Grain Porridge | Berry & Cauliflower Smoothie |
| 18 | Peanut Butter and Jelly Smoothie | Cinnamon Apple Chips with Dip | Pungent Mushroom Barley Risotto | Green Mango Smoothie |

| 19 | Banana Almond Granola | Crunchy Asparagus Spears | Spinach Soup with Dill and Basil | Chia Seed Smoothie |
|---|---|---|---|---|
| 20 | Tasty Oatmeal Muffins | Cucumber Bites with Chive and Sunflower Seeds | Coconut Watercress Soup | Mango Smoothie |
| 21 | Omelet with Chickpea Flour | Garlicky Kale Chips | Coconut Watercress Soup | Fruity Smoothie |

Lightning Source UK Ltd.
Milton Keynes UK
UKHW021017030521
383041UK00001B/34